IT'S THE LAW!

Federal law requires contractors that disturb painted surfaces in homes, child care facilities and schools built before 1978 to be certified and follow specific work practices to prevent lead contamination. Always ask to see your contractor's certification.

Federal law requires that individuals receive certain information before renovating more than six square feet of painted surfaces in a room for interior projects or more than twenty square feet of painted surfaces for exterior projects or window replacement or demolition in housing, child care facilities and schools built before 1978.

- Homeowners and tenants: renovators must give you this pamphlet before starting work.
- Child care facilities, including preschools and kindergarten classrooms, and the families of children under six years of age that attend those facilities: renovators must provide a copy of this pamphlet to child care facilities and general renovation information to families whose children attend those facilities.

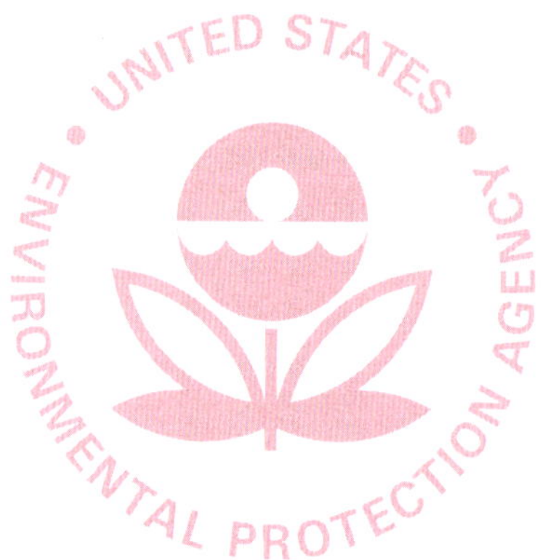

For sale by the Superintendent of Documents, U.S. Government Printing Office
Internet: bookstore.gpo.gov Phone: toll free (866) 512-1800; DC area (202) 512-1800
Fax: (202) 512-2104 Mail: Stop IDCC, Washington. DC 20402-0001

ISBN 978-0-16-090458-5

WHO SHOULD READ THIS PAMPHLET?

This pamphlet is for you if you:

- Reside in a home built before 1978.
- Own or operate a child care facility, including preschools and kindergarten classrooms, built before 1978, or
- Have a child under six years of age who attends a child care facility built before 1978.

You will learn:

- Basic facts about lead and your health.
- How to choose a contractor, if you are a property owner.
- What tenants, and parents/guardians of a child in a child care facility or school should consider.
- How to prepare for the renovation or repair job.
- What to look for during the job and after the job is done.
- Where to get more information about lead.

This pamphlet is not for:

- **Abatement projects.** Abatement is a set of activities aimed specifically at eliminating lead or lead hazards. EPA has regulations for certification and training of abatement professionals. If your goal is to eliminate lead or lead hazards, contact the National Lead Information Center at **1-800-424-LEAD (5323)** for more information.
- **"Do-it-yourself"** projects. If you plan to do renovation work yourself, this document is a good start, but you will need more information to complete the work safely. Call the National Lead Information Center at **1-800-424-LEAD (5323)** and ask for more information on how to work safely in a home with lead-based paint.
- **Contractor education.** Contractors who want information about working safely with lead should contact the National Lead Information Center at **1-800-424-LEAD (5323)** for information about courses and resources on lead-safe work practices.

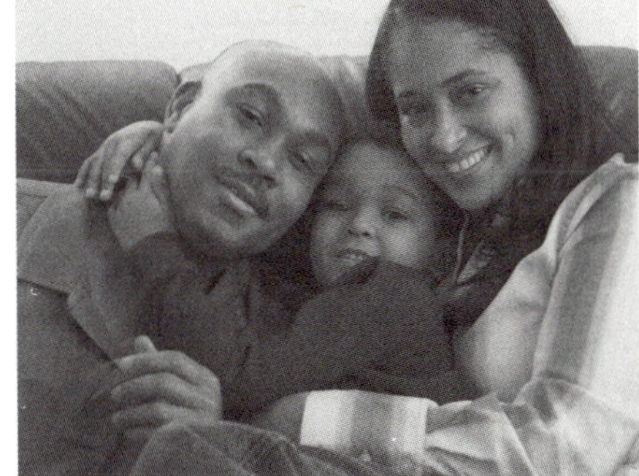

RENOVATING, REPAIRING, OR PAINTING?

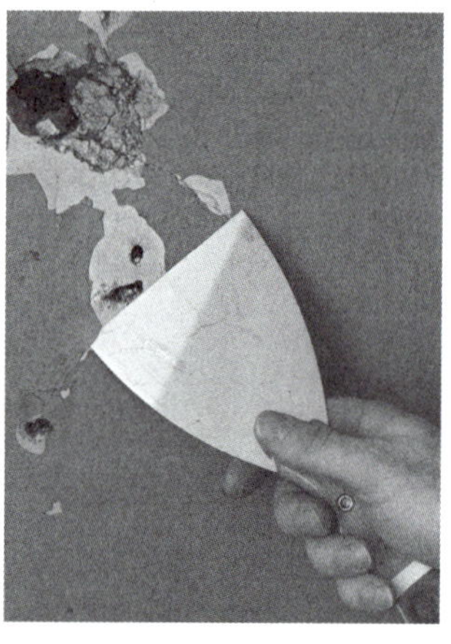

- Is your home, your building, or the child care facility or school your children attend being renovated, repaired, or painted?
- Was your home, your building, or the child care facility or school where your children under six years of age attend built before 1978?

If the answer to these questions is YES, there are a few important things you need to know about lead-based paint.

This pamphlet provides basic facts about lead and information about lead safety when work is being done in your home, your building or the child care facility or school your children attend.

The Facts About Lead

- Lead can affect children's brains and developing nervous systems, causing reduced IQ, learning disabilities, and behavioral problems. Lead is also harmful to adults.
- Lead in dust is the most common way people are exposed to lead. People can also get lead in their bodies from lead in soil or paint chips. Lead dust is often invisible.
- Lead-based paint was used in more than 38 million homes until it was banned for residential use in 1978.
- Projects that disturb painted surfaces can create dust and endanger you and your family. Don't let this happen to you. Follow the practices described in this pamphlet to protect you and your family.

LEAD AND YOUR HEALTH

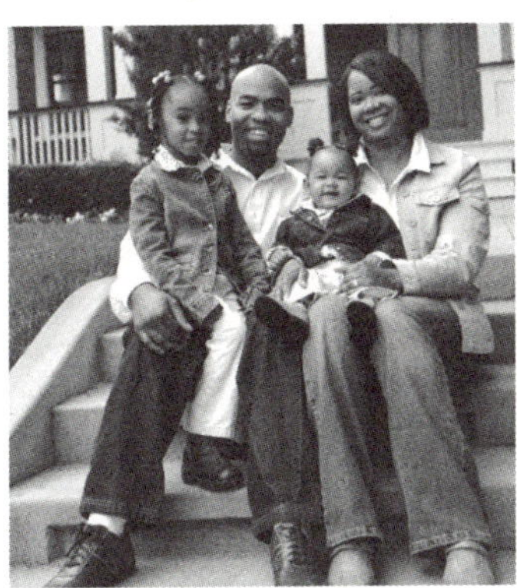

Lead is especially dangerous to children under six years of age.

Lead can affect children's brains and developing nervous systems, causing:

- Reduced IQ and learning disabilities.
- Behavior problems.

Even children who appear healthy can have dangerous levels of lead in their bodies.

Lead is also harmful to adults. In adults, low levels of lead can pose many dangers, including:

- High blood pressure and hypertension.
- Pregnant women exposed to lead can transfer lead to their fetuses. Lead gets into the body when it is swallowed or inhaled.
- People, especially children, can swallow lead dust as they eat, play, and do other normal hand-to-mouth activities.
- People may also breathe in lead dust or fumes if they disturb lead-based paint. People who sand, scrape, burn, brush, blast or otherwise disturb lead-based paint risk unsafe exposure to lead.

What should I do if I am concerned about my family's exposure to lead?

- A blood test is the only way to find out if you or a family member already has lead poisoning. Call your doctor or local health department to arrange for a blood test.
- Call your local health department for advice on reducing and eliminating exposures to lead inside and outside your home, child care facility or school.
- Always use lead-safe work practices when renovation or repair will disturb painted surfaces.

For more information about the health effects of exposure to lead, visit the EPA lead website at **epa.gov/lead/pubs/leadinfo** or call **1-800-424-LEAD (5323)**.

There are other things you can do to protect your family every day.

- Regularly clean floors, window sills, and other surfaces.
- Wash children's hands, bottles, pacifiers, and toys often.
- Make sure children eat a healthy, nutritious diet consistent with the USDA's dietary guidelines, that helps protect children from the effects of lead.
- Wipe off shoes before entering the house.

WHERE DOES THE LEAD COME FROM?

Dust is the main problem.

The most common way to get lead in the body is from dust. Lead dust comes from deteriorating lead-based paint and lead-contaminated soil that gets tracked into your home. This dust may accumulate to unsafe levels. Then, normal hand to-mouth activities, like playing and eating (especially in young children), move that dust from surfaces like floors and window sills into the body.

Home renovation creates dust.

Common renovation activities like sanding, cutting, and demolition can create hazardous lead dust and chips.

Proper work practices protect you from the dust.

The key to protecting yourself and your family during a renovation, repair or painting job is to use lead-safe work practices such as containing dust inside the work area, using dust-minimizing work methods, and conducting a careful cleanup, as described in this pamphlet.

Other sources of lead.

Remember, lead can also come from outside soil, your water, or household items (such as lead-glazed pottery and lead crystal). Contact the National Lead Information Center at **1-800-424-LEAD (5323)** for more information on these sources.

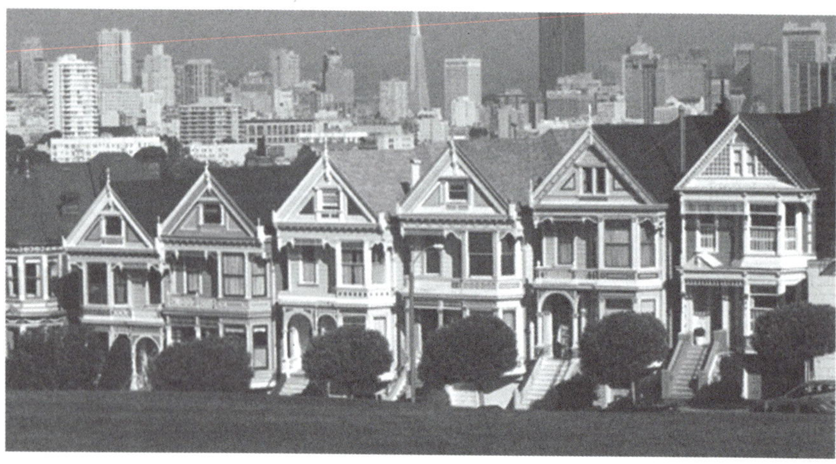

CHECKING YOUR HOME FOR LEAD-BASED PAINT

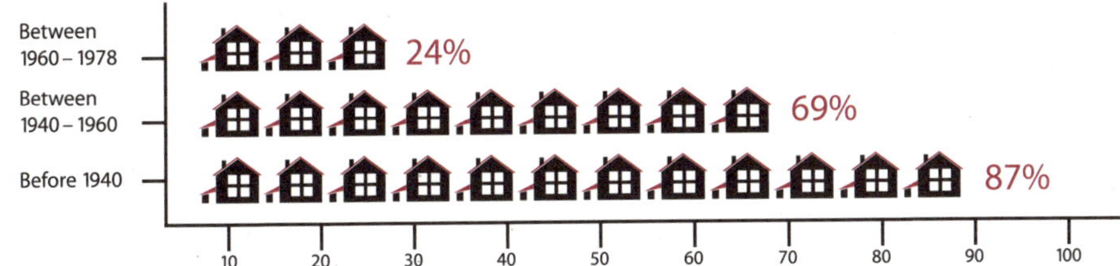

Older homes, child care facilities, and schools are more likely to contain lead-based paint.

Homes may be single-family homes or apartments. They may be private, government-assisted, or public housing. Schools are preschools and kindergarten classrooms. They may be urban, suburban, or rural.

You have the following options:

You may decide to assume your home, child care facility, or school contains lead. Especially in older homes and buildings, you may simply want to assume lead-based paint is present and follow the lead-safe work practices described in this brochure during the renovation, repair, or painting job.

You can hire a certified professional to check for lead-based paint. These professionals are certified risk assessors or inspectors, and can determine if your home has lead or lead hazards.

- A certified inspector or risk assessor can conduct an inspection telling you whether your home, or a portion of your home, has lead-based paint and where it is located. This will tell you the areas in your home where lead-safe work practices are needed.
- A certified risk assessor can conduct a risk assessment telling you if your home currently has any lead hazards from lead in paint, dust, or soil. The risk assessor can also tell you what actions to take to address any hazards.
- For help finding a certified risk assessor or inspector, call the National Lead Information Center at **1-800-424-LEAD (5323)**.

You may also have a certified renovator test the surfaces or components being disturbed for lead by using a lead test kit or by taking paint chip samples and sending them to an EPA-recognized testing laboratory. Test kits must be EPA-recognized and are available at hardware stores. They include detailed instructions for their use.

FOR PROPERTY OWNERS

You have the ultimate responsibility for the safety of your family, tenants, or children in your care.

This means properly preparing for the renovation and keeping persons out of the work area (see p. 8). It also means ensuring the contractor uses lead-safe work practices.

Federal law requires that contractors performing renovation, repair and painting projects that disturb painted surfaces in homes, child care facilities, and schools built before 1978 be certified and follow specific work practices to prevent lead contamination.

Make sure your contractor is certified, and can explain clearly the details of the job and how the contractor will minimize lead hazards during the work.

- You can verify that a contractor is certified by checking EPA's website at **epa.gov/getleadsafe** or by calling the National Lead Information Center at **1-800-424-LEAD (5323)**. You can also ask to see a copy of the contractor's firm certification.
- Ask if the contractor is trained to perform lead-safe work practices and to see a copy of their training certificate.
- Ask them what lead-safe methods they will use to set up and perform the job in your home, child care facility or school.
- Ask for references from at least three recent jobs involving homes built before 1978, and speak to each personally.

Always make sure the contract is clear about how the work will be set up, performed, and cleaned.

- Share the results of any previous lead tests with the contractor.
- You should specify in the contract that they follow the work practices described on pages 9 and 10 of this brochure.
- The contract should specify which parts of your home are part of the work area and specify which lead-safe work practices will be used in those areas. Remember, your contractor should confine dust and debris to the work area and should minimize spreading that dust to other areas of the home.
- The contract should also specify that the contractor will clean the work area, verify that it was cleaned adequately, and re-clean it if necessary.

If you think a worker is not doing what he is supposed to do or is doing something that is unsafe, you should:

- Direct the contractor to comply with regulatory and contract requirements.
- Call your local health or building department, or
- Call EPA's hotline **1-800-424-LEAD (5323)**.

If your property receives housing assistance from HUD (or a state or local agency that uses HUD funds), you must follow the requirements of HUD's Lead-Safe Housing Rule and the ones described in this pamphlet.

FOR TENANTS AND FAMILIES OF CHILDREN UNDER SIX YEARS OF AGE IN CHILD CARE FACILITIES AND SCHOOLS

You play an important role ensuring the ultimate safety of your family.

This means properly preparing for the renovation and staying out of the work area (see p. 8).

Federal law requires that contractors performing renovation, repair and painting projects that disturb painted surfaces in homes built before 1978 and in child care facilities and schools built before 1978, that a child under six years of age visits regularly, to be certified and follow specific work practices to prevent lead contamination.

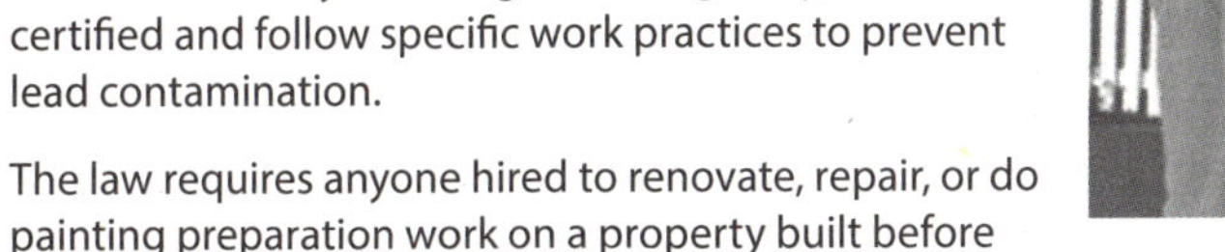

The law requires anyone hired to renovate, repair, or do painting preparation work on a property built before 1978 to follow the steps described on pages 9 and 10 unless the area where the work will be done contains no lead-based paint.

If you think a worker is not doing what he is supposed to do or is doing something that is unsafe, you should:

- Contact your landlord.
- Call your local health or building department, or
- Call EPA's hotline **1-800-424-LEAD (5323)**.

If you are concerned about lead hazards left behind after the job is over, you can check the work yourself (see page 10).

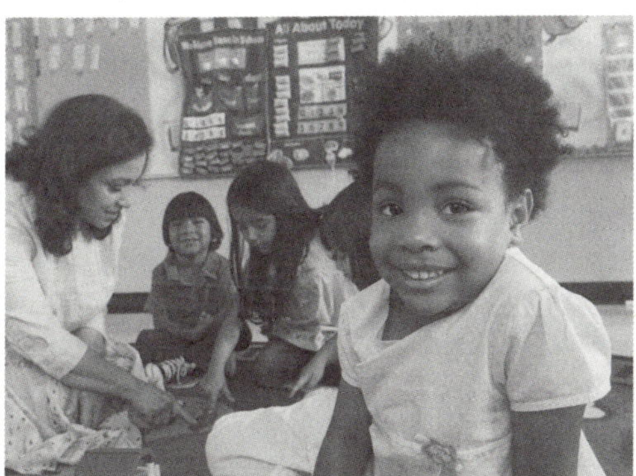

PREPARING FOR A RENOVATION

The work areas should not be accessible to occupants while the work occurs.

The rooms or areas where work is being done may need to be blocked off or sealed with plastic sheeting to contain any dust that is generated. Therefore, the contained area may not be available to you until the work in that room or area is complete, cleaned thoroughly, and the containment has been removed. Because you may not have access to some areas during the renovation, you should plan accordingly.

You may need:

- Alternative bedroom, bathroom, and kitchen arrangements if work is occurring in those areas of your home.
- A safe place for pets because they too can be poisoned by lead and can track lead dust into other areas of the home.
- A separate pathway for the contractor from the work area to the outside in order to bring materials in and out of the home. Ideally, it should not be through the same entrance that your family uses.
- A place to store your furniture. All furniture and belongings may have to be moved from the work area while the work is being done. Items that can't be moved, such as cabinets, should be wrapped in plastic.
- To turn off forced-air heating and air conditioning systems while the work is being done. This prevents dust from spreading through vents from the work area to the rest of your home. Consider how this may affect your living arrangements.

You may even want to move out of your home temporarily while all or part of the work is being done.

Child care facilities and schools may want to consider alternative accommodations for children and access to necessary facilities.

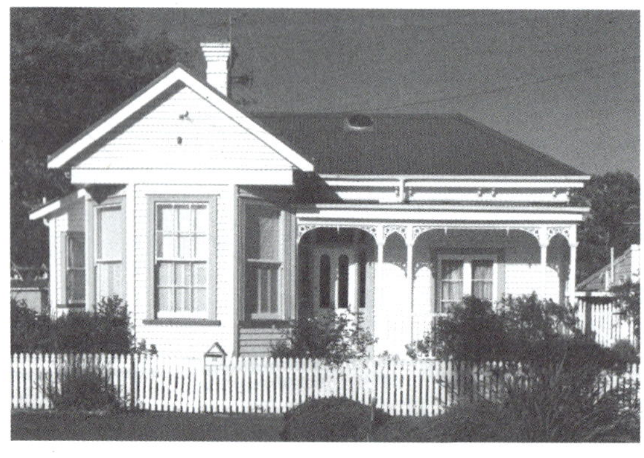

DURING THE WORK

Federal law requires contractors that are hired to perform renovation, repair and painting projects in homes, child care facilities, and schools built before 1978 that disturb painted surfaces to be certified and follow specific work practices to prevent lead contamination.

The work practices the contractor must follow include these three simple procedures, described below:

1. **Contain the work area.** The area must be contained so that dust and debris do not escape from that area. Warning signs must be put up and plastic or other impermeable material and tape must be used as appropriate to:

    - Cover the floors and any furniture that cannot be moved.
    - Seal off doors and heating and cooling system vents.
    - For exterior renovations, cover the ground and, in some instances, erect vertical containment or equivalent extra precautions in containing the work area.

These work practices will help prevent dust or debris from getting outside the work area.

2. **Avoid renovation methods that generate large amounts of lead-contaminated dust.** Some methods generate so much lead-contaminated dust that their use is prohibited. They are:

    - Open flame burning or torching.
    - Sanding, grinding, planing, needle gunning, or blasting with power tools and equipment not equipped with a shroud and HEPA vacuum attachment.
    - Using a heat gun at temperatures greater than 1100°F.

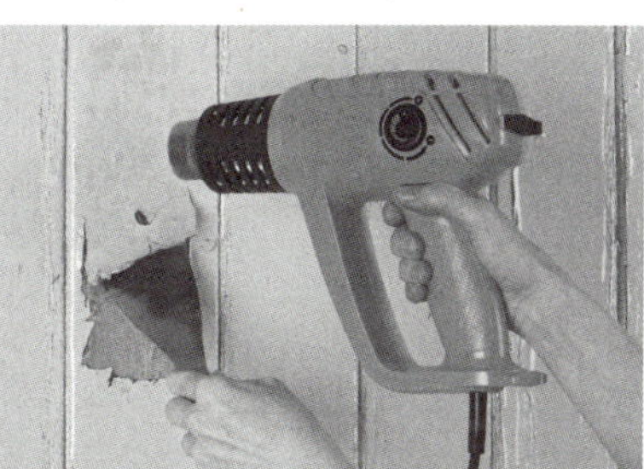

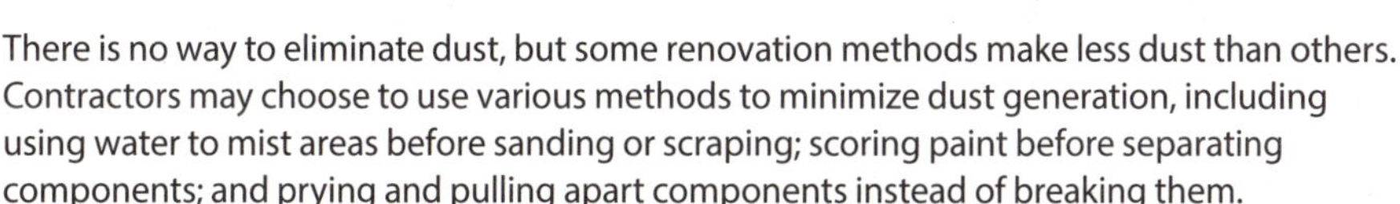

There is no way to eliminate dust, but some renovation methods make less dust than others. Contractors may choose to use various methods to minimize dust generation, including using water to mist areas before sanding or scraping; scoring paint before separating components; and prying and pulling apart components instead of breaking them.

3. **Clean up thoroughly.** The work area should be cleaned up daily to keep it as clean as possible. When all the work is done, the area must be cleaned up using special cleaning methods before taking down any plastic that isolates the work area from the rest of the home. The special cleaning methods should include:

    - Using a HEPA vacuum to clean up dust and debris on all surfaces, followed by
    - Wet wiping and wet mopping with plenty of rinse water.

When the final cleaning is done, look around. There should be no dust, paint chips, or debris in the work area. If you see any dust, paint chips, or debris, the area must be re-cleaned.

FOR PROPERTY OWNERS: AFTER THE WORK IS DONE

When all the work is finished, you will want to know if your home, child care facility, or school where children under six attend has been cleaned up properly.

EPA Requires Cleaning Verification.

In addition to using allowable work practices and working in a lead-safe manner, EPA's RRP rule requires contractors to follow a specific cleaning protocol. The protocol requires the contractor to use disposable cleaning cloths to wipe the floor and other surfaces of the work area and compare these cloths to an EPA-provided cleaning verification card to determine if the work area was adequately cleaned. EPA research has shown that following the use of lead-safe work practices with the cleaning verification protocol will effectively reduce lead-dust hazards.

Lead-Dust Testing.

EPA believes that if you use a certified and trained renovation contractor who follows the LRRP rule by using lead-safe work practices and the cleaning protocol after the job is finished, lead-dust hazards will be effectively reduced. If, however, you are interested in having lead-dust testing done at the completion of your job, outlined below is some helpful information.

What is a lead-dust test?

- Lead-dust tests are wipe samples sent to a laboratory for analysis. You will get a report specifying the levels of lead found after your specific job.

How and when should I ask my contractor about lead-dust testing?

- Contractors are not required by EPA to conduct lead-dust testing. However, if you want testing, EPA recommends testing be conducted by a lead professional. To locate a lead professional who will perform an evaluation near you, visit EPA's website at **epa.gov/lead/pubs/locate** or contact the National Lead Information Center at **1-800-424-LEAD (5323).**

- If you decide that you want lead-dust testing, it is a good idea to specify in your contract, before the start of the job, that a lead-dust test is to be done for your job and who will do the testing, as well as whether re-cleaning will be required based on the results of the test.

- You may do the testing yourself. If you choose to do the testing, some EPA-recognized lead laboratories will send you a kit that allows you to collect samples and send them back to the laboratory for analysis. Contact the National Lead Information Center for lists of EPA-recognized testing laboratories.

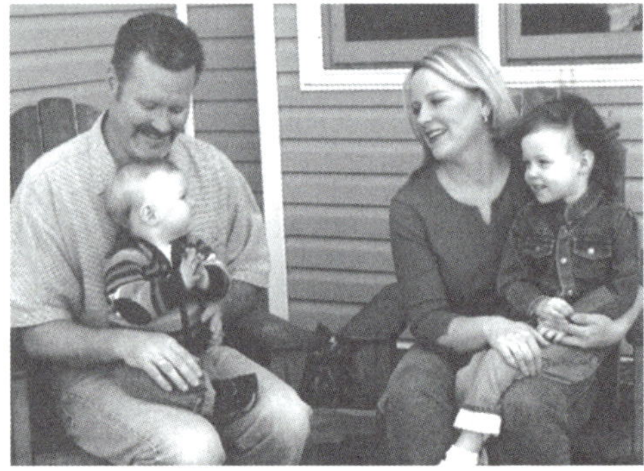

FOR ADDITIONAL INFORMATION

You may need additional information on how to protect yourself and your children while a job is going on in your home, your building, or child care facility.

The National Lead Information Center at **1-800-424-LEAD (5323)** or **epa.gov/lead/nlic** can tell you how to contact your state, local, and/or tribal programs or get general information about lead poisoning prevention.

- State and tribal lead poisoning prevention or environmental protection programs can provide information about lead regulations and potential sources of financial aid for reducing lead hazards. If your state or local government has requirements more stringent than those described in this pamphlet, you must follow those requirements.
- Local building code officials can tell you the regulations that apply to the renovation work that you are planning.
- State, county, and local health departments can provide information about local programs, including assistance for lead-poisoned children and advice on ways to get your home checked for lead.

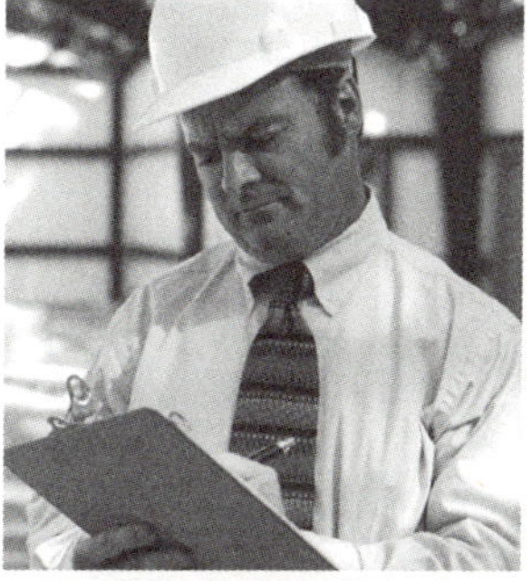

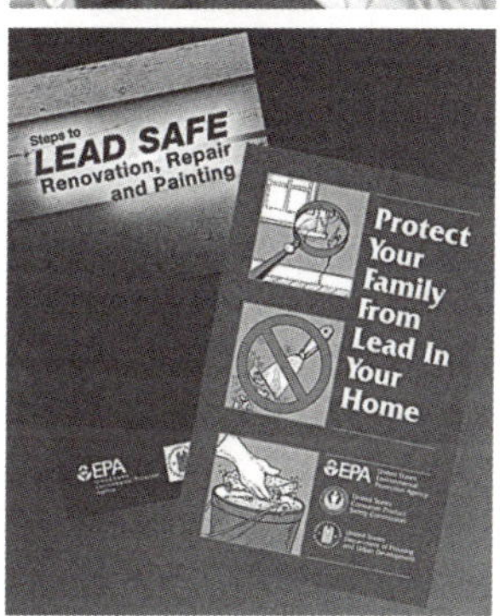

The National Lead Information Center can also provide a variety of resource materials, including the following guides to lead-safe work practices. Many of these materials are also available at **epa.gov/lead/pubs/brochure**

- Steps to Lead Safe Renovation, Repair and Painting.
- Protect Your Family from Lead in Your Home
- Lead in Your Home: A Parent's Reference Guide

For the hearing impaired, call the Federal Information Relay Service at 1-800-877-8339 to access any of the phone numbers in this brochure.

EPA CONTACTS

EPA Regional Offices

EPA addresses residential lead hazards through several different regulations. EPA requires training and certification for conducting abatement and renovations, education about hazards associated with renovations, disclosure about known lead paint and lead hazards in housing, and sets lead-paint hazard standards.

Your Regional EPA Office can provide further information regarding lead safety and lead protection programs at **epa.gov/lead**.

Region 1
(Connecticut, Massachusetts, Maine, New Hampshire, Rhode Island, Vermont)
Regional Lead Contact
U.S. EPA Region 1
Suite 1100
One Congress Street
Boston, MA 02114-2023
(888) 372-7341

Region 2
(New Jersey, New York, Puerto Rico, Virgin Islands)
Regional Lead Contact
U.S. EPA Region 2
2890 Woodbridge Avenue
Building 205, Mail Stop 225
Edison, NJ 08837-3679
(732) 321-6671

Region 3
(Delaware, Maryland, Pennsylvania, Virginia, Washington, DC, West Virginia)
Regional Lead Contact
U.S. EPA Region 3
1650 Arch Street
Philadelphia, PA
19103-2029
(215) 814-5000

Region 4
(Alabama, Florida, Georgia, Kentucky, Mississippi, North Carolina, South Carolina, Tennessee)
Regional Lead Contact
U.S. EPA Region 4
61 Forsyth Street, SW
Atlanta, GA 30303-8960
(404) 562-9900

Region 5
(Illinois, Indiana, Michigan, Minnesota, Ohio, Wisconsin)
Regional Lead Contact
U.S. EPA Region 5
77 West Jackson Boulevard
Chicago, IL 60604-3507
(312) 886-6003

Region 6
(Arkansas, Louisiana, New Mexico, Oklahoma, Texas)
Regional Lead Contact
U.S. EPA Region 6
1445 Ross Avenue,
12th Floor
Dallas, TX 75202-2733
(214) 665-7577

Region 7
(Iowa, Kansas, Missouri, Nebraska)
Regional Lead Contact
U.S. EPA Region 7
901 N. 5th Street
Kansas City, KS 66101
(913) 551-7003

Region 8
(Colorado, Montana, North Dakota, South Dakota, Utah, Wyoming)
Regional Lead Contact
U.S. EPA Region 8
1595 Wynkoop Street
Denver, CO 80202
(303) 312-6312

Region 9
(Arizona, California, Hawaii, Nevada)
Regional Lead Contact
U.S. Region 9
75 Hawthorne Street
San Francisco, CA 94105
(415) 947-8021

Region 10
(Alaska, Idaho, Oregon, Washington)
Regional Lead Contact
U.S. EPA Region 10
1200 Sixth Avenue
Seattle, WA 98101-1128
(206) 553-1200

OTHER FEDERAL AGENCIES

CPSC

The Consumer Product Safety Commission (CPSC) protects the public from the unreasonable risk of injury or death from 15,000 types of consumer products under the agency's jurisdiction. CPSC warns the public and private sectors to reduce exposure to lead and increase consumer awareness. Contact CPSC for further information regarding regulations and consumer product safety.

CPSC
4330 East West Highway
Bethesda, MD 20814
Hotline 1-(800) 638-2772
cpsc.gov

CDC Childhood Lead Poisoning Prevention Branch

The Centers for Disease Control and Prevention (CDC) assists state and local childhood lead poisoning prevention programs to provide a scientific basis for policy decisions, and to ensure that health issues are addressed in decisions about housing and the environment. Contact CDC Childhood Lead Poisoning Prevention Program for additional materials and links on the topic of lead.

CDC Childhood Lead Poisoning Prevention Branch
4770 Buford Highway, MS F-40
Atlanta, GA 30341
(770) 488-3300
cdc.gov/nceh/lead

HUD Office of Healthy Homes and Lead Hazard Control

The Department of Housing and Urban Development (HUD) provides funds to state and local governments to develop cost-effective ways to reduce lead-based paint hazards in America's privately-owned low-income housing. In addition, the office enforces the rule on disclosure of known lead paint and lead hazards in housing, and HUD's lead safety regulations in HUD-assisted housing, provides public outreach and technical assistance, and conducts technical studies to help protect children and their families from health and safety hazards in the home. Contact the HUD Office of Healthy Homes and Lead Hazard Control for information on lead regulations, outreach efforts, and lead hazard control research and outreach grant programs.

U.S. Department of Housing and Urban Development
Office of Healthy Homes and
Lead Hazard Control
451 Seventh Street, SW, Room 8236
Washington, DC 20410-3000
HUD's Lead Regulations Hotline
(202) 402-7698
hud.gov/offices/lead/

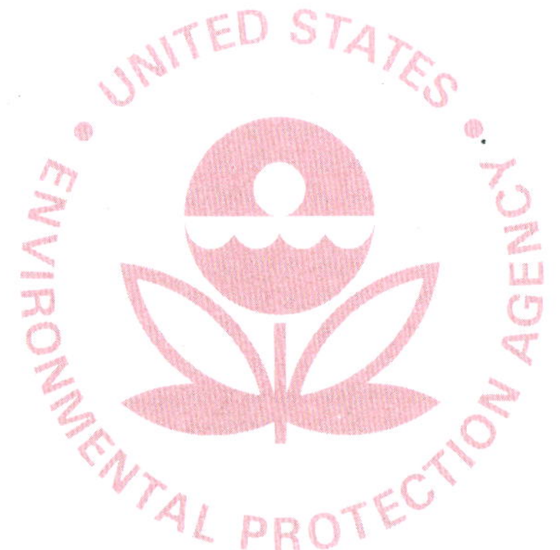
UNITED STATES
ENVIRONMENTAL PROTECTION AGENCY

SAMPLE PRE-RENOVATION FORM

This sample form may be used by renovation firms to document compliance with the Federal pre-renovation education and renovation, repair, and painting regulations.

Occupant Confirmation

Pamphlet Receipt

❑ I have received a copy of the lead hazard information pamphlet informing me of the potential risk of the lead hazard exposure from renovation activity to be performed in my dwelling unit. I received this pamphlet before the work began.

____

Printed Name of Owner-occupant

______________________ ______________________

Signature of Owner-occupant Signature Date

Renovator's Self Certification Option (for tenant-occupied dwellings only)

Instructions to Renovator: If the lead hazard information pamphlet was delivered but a tenant signature was not obtainable, you may check the appropriate box below.

❑ **Declined** – I certify that I have made a good faith effort to deliver the lead hazard information pamphlet to the rental dwelling unit listed below at the date and time indicated and that the occupant declined to sign the confirmation of receipt. I further certify that I have left a copy of the pamphlet at the unit with the occupant.

❑ **Unavailable for signature** – I certify that I have made a good faith effort to deliver the lead hazard information pamphlet to the rental dwelling unit listed below and that the occupant was unavailable to sign the confirmation of receipt. I further certify that I have left a copy of the pamphlet at the unit by sliding it under the door or by (fill in how pamphlet was left).

______________________ ______________________

Printed Name of Person Certifying Delivery Attempted Delivery Date

____

Signature of Person Certifying Lead Pamphlet Delivery

____

____

____

Unit Address

Note Regarding Mailing Option — As an alternative to delivery in person, you may mail the ead hazard information pamphlet to the owner and/or tenant. Pamphlet must be mailed at east seven days before renovation. Mailing must be documented by a certificate of mailing 'rom the post office.